The Art of Compassionate Living:

Simple Habits for Holistic Health

DR. TINILLE T. JENKINS, DMS, PA-C

Foreword By: Dr. Kim Callwood, MD

Dr. Of Radiology

The Art of Compassionate Living
Simple Habits for Holistic Health

Library of Congress Control Number: 2024910209

ISBN: 979-8-9900951-1-3

Published by: JTI
Bowie, MD. 20721

ttj@jtillc.com

Editor: Dr. Joseph Amanfu
Cover Design & Illustration: JTI
Interior Design: JTI

Printed in the USA

Disclaimer: This book is intended to provide accurate information in regard to the subject matter covered. All information is deemed accurate; however, it is for educational purposes only. The reader is advised to seek professional services for their unique situation.

Dedication

This book is lovingly dedicated to the pillars of my strength and the keepers of my heart:

To my Mom, Tina, and Dad, Willis, whose unwavering support has been my anchor in every storm and joy. To Tenise, Kynze, and Trent, who have been my steadfast companions on this journey, always encouraging me as I reach higher and for bigger dreams.

To my maternal grandparents, Aretha and the memory of Tillman Frizzell, Jr., and the memory of my paternal grandparents, Dorothy and Willis Jenkins, Sr., whose legacies of resilience and love continue to guide me. To the memory of my great aunt Jeanne, and my great aunt and uncle, Eudelle and James, as well as great uncle Wilson, whose prayers have upheld me and whose love has fortified me.

To my extended family and all those I hold dear as family, thank you for enveloping me in love and lifting me with your prayers. This achievement is not just mine, but a reflection of your faith in me and the collective hope we share.

Who Should Read This Book?

I wrote **The Art of Compassionate Living** to promote compassion as a way of living and as part of my legacy of promoting healthy living by doing the following **CPR**:

1. **C**hoosing Love over Hate

2. **P**roviding Kindness Often

3. **R**eaffirming the Broken Hearted

This CPR acrostic beautifully **illuminates the life-saving and transformative power of compassion in our lives and relationships. If this can be your mission, then this book is for you.**

My Desire: To have **you** and as many as will perform CPR. CPR or Cardiopulmonary Resuscitation is **an emergency lifesaving procedure performed when the heart stops beating...**

1. Choosing Love Over Hate is like CPR for the Soul

Imagine someone's heart just stopped. That's a crisis, right? CPR is what we do to jump-start the heart, to bring someone back from the edge. Now, think about a world that's often cold and harsh, filled with hate and indifference. Choosing love over hate in such a world is like being that person who jumps in to do CPR. It's about refusing to let the coldness win, pumping warmth and life back into our surroundings with every choice we make. It's an act of bravery, a decision to fight against the tide of negativity, keeping the pulse of humanity strong with love.

2. Providing Kindness Often Keeps the Blood Flowing Think of kindness as the chest compressions in CPR. Just as compressions keep the blood flowing, keeping the person alive until help arrives, our acts of kindness keep the spirit of our communities alive. It's all about consistency. One act of kindness can be powerful, but when we're kind often, it's like those steady compressions on a chest, absolutely vital. It keeps hope alive, it keeps the connection alive, and it reminds everyone around that goodness hasn't left the building. It's about making kindness a rhythm, a heartbeat that everyone can dance to.

3. Reaffirming the Broken Hearted is like Giving Breath
In the tender act of consoling the broken-hearted, we do more than share words; we breathe hope into their world. Think of it as filling their lungs with hope, letting them breathe in a sense of belonging and breathe out the pain and isolation. It's a profound embrace that says, "You're not alone." Such moments fill the soul with belonging and ease the weight of solitude. This shared strength is the essence of compassion; it's our collective heartbeat, reviving the spirit of hope and ensuring no one is left out in the cold. Compassion, like CPR for the heart, is a life skill that demands practice and a generous heart.

FOREWORD

In an era that often feels dominated by divisiveness and indifference, the timeless virtues of empathy and kindness stand out as beacons of hope, guiding us toward a more compassionate society. *The Art of Compassionate Living*, penned by Tinille Jenkins, serves as both a mirror and a map: reflecting our deepest values back to us and charting a course toward personal growth and societal healing. Tinille, known for her innate compassion and dedication to healthcare, infuses each page with insights drawn from her own experiences as a tireless advocate for kindness.

At the heart of Tinille's approach to compassionate living is the understanding that every interaction is an opportunity to enrich our own lives as well as those of others. Whether it's offering a listening ear, extending a helping hand, or simply sharing a moment of understanding, these actions build bridges of empathy that can span seemingly insurmountable divides. Through practical advice and inspiring stories, Tinille provides the tools needed to transform compassion from a mere concept into a daily practice.

As you explore the pages of this book, you'll find yourself deeply moved by Tinille Jenkins' personal stories and the broader tales of kindness she shares. Each one shines a light on what we can achieve at our best compassion, connection, and genuine care for each other. These stories aren't just heartwarming; they're powerful calls to action, reminding us that every day gives us a new chance to be part of a greater legacy of kindness. Allow Tinille to lead you on a transformative journey of personal growth and meaningful contributions to society, where you'll learn to apply the power of compassion in all areas of your life.

Dr. Kim Callwood, MD.
Doctor of Radiology

Table of Contents

Acknowledgments

This book is a testament not only to my personal journey but also to the extraordinary circle of support that has surrounded me. I am profoundly grateful to each and every one of you.

To my mom, Tina, whose encouragement and guidance were instrumental in the creation of this work. Your wisdom and love have been the bedrock upon which I built my dreams. To my dad, Willis, and my loving sister, Tenise, thank you for being the most engaging and supportive study partners I could ever wish for. You made the arduous path to reaching my goals possible and shared the journey.

To my maternal grandmother, Rea, whose presence in my life has been a constant source of comfort and care. Thank you for being there at every turn, making each new apartment feel like home with your weeks-long visits and nurturing spirit. To Dr. Kim, who demystified the world of medicine for me and made all things medical make sense.

Special thanks to Lauren, PA-C, for your prayers and words of encouragement when I needed them most. To Pastor Brenda, Elder Helen, and Uncle Paul, for being the prayer warrior leaders in my faith community and your unwavering faith and prayers have been a guiding light in my spiritual and personal growth. To Dr. Meixer, who has been cheering me on since my undergraduate days, your support has never wavered and so many letters of recommendations mailed on my behalf.

To Michael, for your thoughtful presence in my life, always understanding and supportive. To Denice, Jade, Kynze, Ronnie, Sean, and many others (you know who you are) for each conversation with me that brought me closer to yet another graduation, another milestone.

This book is because of all of you. Your collective support, love, and belief in my abilities have brought me to this incredible point in my life, allowing me to share my journey and insights. From the bottom of my heart, thank you for being part of my story.

Words from the Author

These pages are filled with a simple yet profound hope: that the words you find here serve not just as a guide but as a spark— a catalyst for transformation both within you and in the ripples, you create around you. Each chapter, though brief, is crafted with care to nudge your heart, challenge your perspectives, and inspire action. It's not just about understanding compassion; it's about living it, breathing it into every nook of your existence. There are exercises at the end of each chapter. Why? They're your toolkit, your practice ground. Like seeds planted in fertile soil, they have the potential to grow to blossom into actions and habits that not only enrich your life but also touch the lives of others.

Think of this book as a conversation, one that I hope will continue long after you turn the last page. It's an invitation to pause, reflect, and step boldly into a compassion-driven journey. And remember, the true beauty of this journey lies not in the grand gestures but in the quiet moments, the small acts of kindness, the gentle words of understanding. These are the moments that weave together to form a tapestry of profound change. So, as you embark on this path, know that every step taken in compassion is a step towards a more loving, empathetic world. I say, "Empathy and Care, Wellness Everywhere." Let's walk this path together, shall we?

Chapter 1

MINDFUL AWARENESS

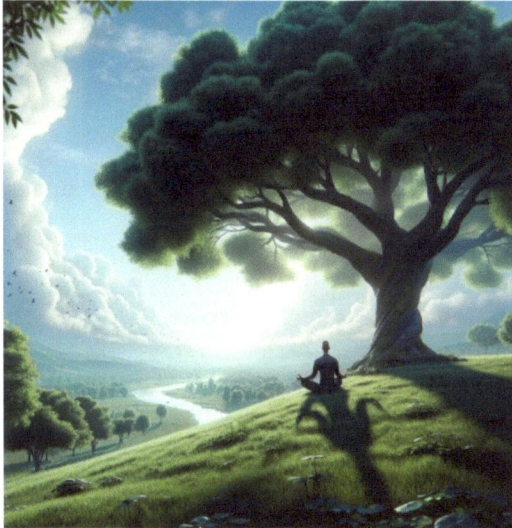

Mindful Awareness

"True relationships are nurtured with patience, kindness, and the willingness to understand each other's journey."
~ *Karen A. Baquiran*

Mindfulness is the practice of intentionally focusing one's attention on the present moment and accepting it without judgment. It involves being fully aware of our thoughts, feelings, bodily sensations, and the surrounding environment, allowing us to observe our experiences without being caught up in them. This practice encourages a state of open, nonjudgmental awareness, enabling individuals to engage more fully with life as it unfolds moment by moment. Mindfulness has its roots in ancient meditation practices, but it's also a secular and practical approach to enhancing mental and emotional well-being, fostering greater clarity, calm, and insight in daily life. To simplify, let me share a story:

Once, in a tranquil village nestled among lush forests and serene rivers, lived a wise elder known for her remarkable tranquility and insight. Despite the village's usual bustle and occasional strife, she moved through her days with a calm grace that intrigued those around her. One day, a young villager, burdened by the weight of her worries and the relentless pace of life, approached the elder seeking guidance. "How do you find peace amid chaos?" she asked. The elder invited the young woman to sit beside her under a sprawling oak tree, handing her a smooth, round stone. "Hold this," she said, "and for a few moments, just observe it. Notice its weight, its temperature, its texture."

As the young woman did so, her mind began to quiet. The concerns that had seemed so pressing began to fade, replaced by a simple awareness of the stone in her hand. "This," the elder explained, "is mindfulness. It's the art of being wholly present with whatever is before you, whether a stone, a task, or a moment of your life. It doesn't erase life's challenges, but it changes how you experience them. You learn to meet each moment with presence and kindness towards yourself and others." The young woman felt a shift within her, a glimpse of the elder's peace. She realized that mindfulness wasn't a destination but a path, one that she could walk every day, one present moment at a time. From that day forward, the young villager practiced mindfulness in her daily activities, finding in it a wellspring of peace and compassion. As she shared this practice with others, the entire village began to transform, embodying a collective calm that mirrored the tranquility of their wise elder. Through mindfulness, they discovered not just the joy of being present but the profound connection it fostered within themselves and their community.

Mindfulness Introduction:

Embarking on a journey through mindful awareness, this chapter gently introduces the concept of mindfulness, a compassionate and reflective practice central to nurturing a deeper understanding of oneself and the world around us. Particularly for young women forging paths in their careers, mindfulness offers a sanctuary from the whirlwind of daily commitments and challenges. It teaches the art of being present, cultivating an inner space of calm and clarity amid life's storms. Through embracing mindfulness, you're not just learning to navigate your professional and personal landscapes with grace but also fostering an environment where compassion towards oneself and others flourishes.

This chapter lays the foundation for a transformative practice that promises to enhance every facet of your being, illuminating the richness of the present moment and empowering you to approach your aspirations with a heart full of compassion.

The Practice of Mindful Awareness

The practice of mindful awareness is akin to learning a new language, the language of your own mind and body. It involves a series of simple yet profound techniques that guide you to tune in to your present experiences with openness and curiosity. One foundational technique is mindful breathing, where you focus your attention solely on the rhythm of your breath, its natural flow in and out of your body, allowing thoughts and distractions to pass by without engagement, like clouds drifting across the sky. Another technique involves a body scan, where you mentally traverse through different parts of your body, noticing any sensations, tension, or comfort without judgment. This not only cultivates awareness but also fosters a deep connection with the physical self. Mindful walking is yet another practice, transforming ordinary walks into meditative journeys by concentrating on the sensation of each step, the feel of the ground under your feet, and the rhythm of your movement. Each of these practices serves as a tool to anchor you in the present, creating a space where you can observe your thoughts, feelings, and physical sensations with detachment and kindness. By regularly engaging in these practices, you develop the ability to remain present and attentive, even amidst the chaos of daily life, nurturing a state of calm and clarity that enriches both your personal and professional worlds.

Benefits for Health

The benefits of mindful awareness for both emotional and physical well-being are profound and well-documented. Emotionally, mindfulness acts as a grounding force, reducing stress, anxiety, and depressive symptoms by fostering a state of calm and acceptance. It teaches practitioners to observe their thoughts and emotions without being overwhelmed by them, promoting a healthier psychological state. This enhanced emotional regulation can lead to improved relationships, increased resilience, and a greater sense of inner peace. Physically, the benefits are equally significant. Regular mindfulness practice has been linked to lower blood pressure, improved sleep, and a stronger immune system. It can also alleviate chronic pain by changing the way pain is perceived, making it more manageable. Furthermore, mindfulness encourages healthier lifestyle choices, as increased body awareness often leads to better eating habits and more regular exercise. In essence, mindful awareness cultivates holistic well-being, harmonizing the mind and body and paving the way for a life lived with greater health, happiness, and harmony.

Mindful awareness emerges as a transformative practice, guiding us to experience life with deeper clarity and compassion. By embracing mindfulness through practices like mindful breathing and body scans, we learn to navigate life's complexities with greater ease, fostering both emotional and physical well-being. This chapter reveals mindfulness as more than a coping mechanism; it's a pathway to living more authentically, offering profound benefits from reduced stress to enhanced health and deeper connections. As we journey through mindfulness, each moment becomes an opportunity for discovery and growth, encouraging us to live with intention and embrace the richness of the present. This is your invitation to begin a transformative journey, one mindful moment at a time.

Take Action: Mindful Awareness Exercise

Reflective Exercise:

For beginners looking to weave mindful awareness into the fabric of their daily lives, starting with a simple, reflective exercise can be immensely beneficial. Begin each day with a five-minute mindfulness meditation. Sit in a comfortable position in a quiet space, close your eyes, and focus on your breath. Pay attention to the sensation of air entering and leaving your body, the rise and fall of your chest, and any sounds or sensations around you. When your mind wanders, as it inevitably will, gently acknowledge the thought and then bring your focus back to your breath. This practice helps in cultivating a moment-to-moment awareness, anchoring you in the present. Throughout the day, take short "mindfulness breaks." Pause for a minute or two to observe your surroundings and the texture of your immediate experience, or simply return your attention to your breath. These brief interludes can act as resets, reducing stress and enhancing clarity. Lastly, end your day with a gratitude exercise. Reflect on three things you were grateful for that day, however big or small. This not only fosters a positive mindset but also deepens your mindfulness practice by encouraging you to notice and appreciate the simple joys of daily life. By integrating these exercises into your routine, you embark on a journey of mindful living, gradually cultivating a deeper awareness and appreciation for the present moment.

This not only fosters a positive mindset but also deepens your mindfulness practice by encouraging you to notice and appreciate the simple joys of daily life. By integrating these exercises into your routine, you embark on a journey of mindful living, gradually cultivating a deeper awareness and appreciation for the present moment.

Chapter 2

SELF-COMPASSION

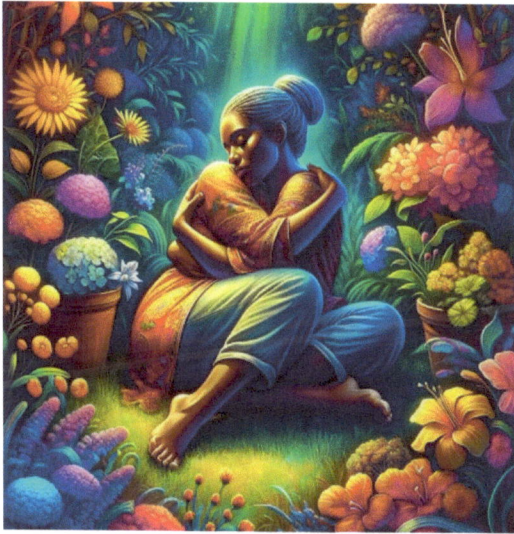

SELF-COMPASSION

"In the stillness of mindful awareness, we discover the profound depths of our own being, where peace and clarity reside"
~ Jon Kabat-Zinn

Self-compassion is a gentle yet powerful practice of treating oneself with kindness, understanding, and acceptance, especially during times of difficulty or failure. It involves three core elements: self-kindness, which encourages a nurturing attitude towards oneself; common humanity, which recognizes that suffering and imperfection are universal experiences; and mindfulness, which allows us to observe our thoughts and feelings without judgment. Embracing self-compassion leads to increased resilience, improved mental health, and a more compassionate and fulfilling relationship with oneself and others. It's a transformative approach that shifts how we relate to ourselves, fostering a kind, connected, and mindful presence through life's ups and downs.

I believe you can imagine that pursuing my rigorous academic journey of becoming a Physician Associate (PA) required the three aforementioned core elements of self-compassion to graduate with my sanity. I recognized the strain I was under. Constantly pushing through the demanding curriculum, I seldom took moments to pause and appreciate my own hard work and accomplishments. This realization prompted me to make a crucial decision about self-care and self-compassion. Deciding to reward myself for my educational strides, I planned a much-needed getaway to Puerto Rico, a place I hadn't visited in years. Despite the constraints of a student budget and the limited time I could spare, I was determined to make the trip happen. With some financial help from my parents, for which I was grateful, I managed to arrange an abrupt and short vacation. Often times it is okay to accept help from your support system. ☺

Accompanied by my mother, I set off for Puerto Rico, eager to immerse myself in its sunny weather and stunning landscapes. The escape to this beautiful island was not just about taking a break but about honoring my efforts and achievements in a tangible way. We stayed close to the vibrant shores, allowing the soothing sounds of the ocean to wash away the academic lifestyle, and the peace outside of classroom walls began to consume me.

One of the highlights of our trip was visiting El Yunque National Forest. The lush greenery and the serene environment felt miles away from the hectic pace of academia. We also explored Old San Juan, captivated by its rich history and picturesque scenery. The colorful buildings and cobblestone streets were a delightful feast for the senses.

This vacation was not merely a break from routine but a vital part of my journey towards embracing self-compassion. It served as a healthy reset, rejuvenating both my mind and spirit. The experience reinforced the importance of taking time for oneself, especially amidst life's relentless demands.

Through this journey, I learned that practicing self-compassion is as crucial as any academic endeavor. It's about acknowledging your hard work, allowing yourself to enjoy your successes, and understanding that seeking help and taking breaks are not signs of weakness but acts of strength.

Reflecting on this trip, I am reminded of the power of self-care and the profound impact it can have on one's well-being. It has taught me to be kinder to myself and to make self-compassion a regular part of my life, not just as a student but in my future career and personal life as well.

Understanding Self-Compassion

The heart of self-compassion, unraveling its components and illuminating its significance in our lives can be challenging. Self-compassion is founded on three key elements: kindness towards oneself, recognition of our common humanity, and mindfulness. It teaches us to treat ourselves with the same kindness and understanding we would offer a good friend, especially in times of failure or difficulty. This nurturing attitude allows us to acknowledge our imperfections without harsh judgment, understanding that mistakes and setbacks are universal aspects of the human experience. By embracing self-compassion, we foster a resilient and

12

caring relationship with ourselves, paving the way for personal growth, improved mental health, and a more fulfilling life. Recognizing the value of self-compassion is transformative; it acts as a foundation for building self-worth and navigating life's challenges with grace and resilience, marking a pivotal step toward holistic well-being.

Overcoming Self-Criticism

Overcoming self-criticism involves intentional strategies to shift from a mindset of harsh judgment to one of kindness and support. A key strategy is recognizing and challenging negative self-talk. This can be achieved by first becoming aware of the critical inner voice and then questioning its accuracy and helpfulness. Replacing critical thoughts with more compassionate and constructive messages is vital. Practicing affirmations that emphasize personal strengths and values can reinforce a positive self-image. Another effective approach is to imagine what a supportive friend would say in challenging moments and to offer those words to oneself. Mindfulness plays a crucial role here, as it helps to observe thoughts without attachment, allowing negative self-talk to pass through without internalizing it. Cultivating a kinder internal dialogue is not about denying difficulties but about approaching them with understanding and compassion, which fosters resilience and healthier self-esteem.

Benefits for Mental Health

Self-compassion plays a transformative role in mental health, acting as a buffer against anxiety, depression, and stress. By fostering an attitude of kindness and understanding towards oneself, individuals can navigate life's challenges with greater ease and resilience. Self-compassion encourages a gentle acknowledgment of one's feelings and experiences without over-identification, which helps in reducing the intensity of negative emotions and thoughts. This approach diminishes the impact of stressors by promoting a balanced perspective and preventing the spiral of negative self-evaluation that often exacerbates mental health issues. Research has consistently shown that those who practice self-compassion experience lower levels of anxiety and depression, as they are better equipped to cope with difficult situations and feelings. Moreover, self-compassion nurtures emotional resilience, empowering individuals to bounce back from setbacks with a sense of understanding and forgiveness toward themselves. In essence, self-compassion is not just a practice but a pathway to a more peaceful and resilient state of mind, offering profound benefits for mental health and well-being.

As we wrap up this journey into understanding and embracing self-compassion has unfolded as a transformative process essential for nurturing our mental and emotional well-being. We've explored the components of self-compassion, its significance, and practical strategies for overcoming self-criticism, along with the profound benefits it holds for mental health. Through reflective exercises like writing a compassionate letter to oneself, we've seen how cultivating a kinder internal dialogue can lead to increased resilience, reduced anxiety, and a deeper sense of peace and self-acceptance. This chapter invited us to shift our perspective, encouraging us to treat ourselves with the same empathy and understanding we would offer a close friend. Embracing self-compassion is a courageous step towards healing, growth, and unlocking a more compassionate, fulfilled life. It's a journey well worth embarking on as we learn to become our own best ally in the face of life's challenges.

Take Action: Write Your Compassion Letter

Reflective Exercise: Writing a Letter to Oneself

Purpose: Cultivate self-compassion through understanding and kindness.

Method: Address the letter to yourself as you would to a dear friend.

Contents:

- Acknowledge personal struggles and validate your feelings.
- Offer words of encouragement and support for challenges faced.
- Highlight personal strengths and efforts made.
- Remind yourself of your inherent worth and the commonality of imperfection and growth.

Benefits:

- Serves as a tangible reminder of a compassionate stance towards oneself.
- Helps internalize a loving and forgiving inner dialogue.
- Confronts self-criticism and replaces it with a nurturing voice.
- Reinforces the belief in deserving the same kindness and care offered to others.
- Deepens the relationship with oneself, fostering resilience and a compassionate heart.

Chapter 3

GRATITUDE PRACTICE

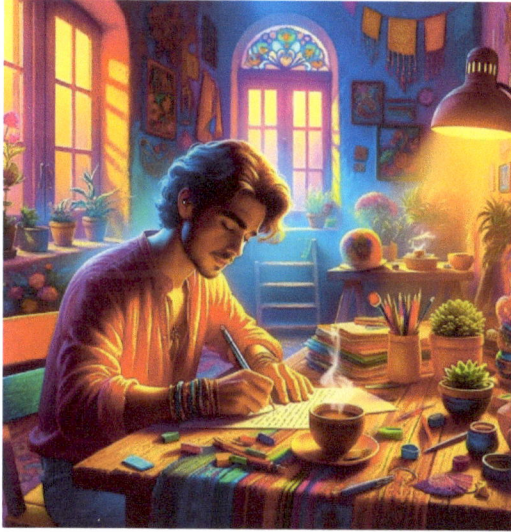

Gratitude Practice

Gratitude practice is a transformative and enriching habit that nurtures joy, resilience, and connection in our lives. It involves recognizing and appreciating the value in everything around us, from the grand to the mundane. This intentional focus on the positive aspects of our existence can significantly boost our mental and emotional well-being, foster deeper relationships, and enhance our overall sense of satisfaction with life. By adopting simple practices, such as maintaining a gratitude journal or sharing expressions of thankfulness with others, we cultivate a mindset that appreciates the present and acknowledges the abundance in our lives. Gratitude practice is a key to unlocking a more contented, connected, and joyful journey through life.

In my life, the practice of gratitude has become a vital source of strength and joy, particularly through the daily ritual of meditation. During these moments of quiet reflection, I engage deeply with my thoughts and focus on visualizing moments that evoke a profound sense of gratefulness.

One of the most cherished series of memories that I often return to during my meditation involves the times I spent with my maternal grandparents. These memories are not just mere recollections; they are vivid experiences that continue to enrich my life and enhance my gratitude practice.

For example, I remember distinctly the sounds and sensations associated with my grandmother's visits during my years in academia. Her presence was a comforting constant in my otherwise hectic life. She traveled multiple times just to be with me, each visit a testament to her unwavering love and support. I can still recall the aroma of the meals she cooked, which filled my small student apartment, transforming it into a space of warmth and familiarity. We would watch movies together, an activity that not only entertained us but also strengthened our bond. Her willingness to perform everyday activities with me, like grocery shopping, was imbued with such tenderness and care that even the most mundane tasks became special. Most importantly, her hugs—offered generously and just when I needed them most—were a sanctuary of comfort and love.

Similarly, my memories with my grandfather are filled with warmth and laughter, especially those quiet times spent on the couch watching his favorite sports teams. His enthusiasm was infectious, and his joy became mine. During the games, he would often pull me into a tight hug, a simple gesture that conveyed so much love and reassurance.

Through meditation, these moments become more than just memories; they are vivid, living experiences that I carry forward into my present. Each session not only allows me to relive these times but also deepens my appreciation for the profound impact my grandparents had on my life.

This practice of gratitude through visualization not only nurtures my emotional well-being but also reinforces my connections with those I love, transcending time and space. It teaches me that gratitude is not just about acknowledging the good in life but also about recognizing the sources of this goodness and the ways they continue to influence and support me.

In sharing this narrative, I hope to inspire others to explore their own gratitude practice. By finding time to reflect on and appreciate the relationships and moments that have shaped us, we can cultivate a deeper sense of fulfillment and peace in our lives.

The Power of Gratitude

Let's unveil the transformative power of gratitude, a simple yet profound practice with far-reaching effects on mental and emotional health. Gratitude goes beyond mere appreciation; it's an active acknowledgment of the good in our lives, often leading to a shift in how we perceive our circumstances. This shift fosters a positive outlook, diminishing the impact of negative emotions and enhancing well-being. Studies have shown that individuals who regularly practice gratitude experience lower levels of stress and depression, as focusing on positive aspects helps counterbalance the brain's natural tendency to dwell on threats or worries. Moreover, gratitude strengthens social bonds and self-esteem, creating a sense of connectedness and increased satisfaction with life. By integrating gratitude into daily routines—whether through journaling, meditation, or verbal expressions—we nurture a resilient, joy-filled perspective, grounding ourselves in the present and opening our hearts to a fuller appreciation of life's gifts.

Cultivating a Gratitude Mindset

Cultivating a gratitude mindset involves intentional practices that steer the mind towards recognizing and appreciating the abundance present in our lives, even in the midst of challenges. A practical and effective method is maintaining a gratitude journal, where daily entries of things you're thankful for can significantly uplift your mood and perspective. This could range from simple joys like a warm cup of coffee to profound aspects such as the support of loved ones. Another tip is to start or end your day by reflecting on three things you are grateful for, which primes your brain to notice the positive. Integrating gratitude into your conversations by sharing what you're thankful for with others not only amplifies your feelings of gratitude but also fosters a positive environment around you. Mindfulness practices, such as mindful walks where you appreciate the beauty in your surroundings, can deepen your sense of gratitude by connecting you more closely to the present moment.

Cultivating a gratitude mindset isn't about ignoring life's difficulties but about balancing your view to include the good with the bad, leading to a more fulfilled and emotionally resilient life.

Benefits for Relationships:

The practice of gratitude has a remarkable ability to strengthen connections and deepen relationships through the power of shared appreciation. When we express gratitude towards others, it not only acknowledges their positive impact on our lives but also reinforces their value and our appreciation for them. This act of recognition fosters mutual respect and affection, enhancing the bond between individuals. Gratitude encourages a cycle of generosity and kindness, as those who feel appreciated are more likely to express their own gratitude and kindness in return, creating a positive feedback loop within relationships. Furthermore, shared gratitude experiences, such as verbalizing what you're thankful for about each other or writing appreciation notes, enhance communication and understanding, leading to stronger, more resilient connections. By making gratitude a regular part of interactions, relationships flourish under a culture of appreciation and empathy, paving the way for deeper, more meaningful connections that withstand the test of time.

In closing, the exploration of gratitude's power reveals its profound impact on enhancing mental and emotional health, cultivating a positive mindset, and fortifying relationships through shared appreciation. Embracing gratitude in daily life, from maintaining a gratitude journal to expressing thankfulness in interactions, transforms our perspective, encouraging us to focus on the abundance and goodness that surround us. This practice not only enriches our personal well-being but also radiates outward, strengthening our connections with others by fostering a culture of appreciation and mutual respect. Gratitude, therefore, is not just an act of recognition but a transformative force capable of deepening our joy, resilience, and sense of connectedness in an ever-complex world. By integrating gratitude into our daily routines, we open our hearts to a more fulfilling, compassionate, and appreciative way of living.

Take Action: Gratitude Journaling

Reflective Exercise: Keeping a Gratitude Journal

Purpose: Foster a gratitude mindset and enhance overall well-being.

- Method: Make daily entries of things you are thankful for.
- Suggestions for Entries:
  - Simple pleasures (e.g., a peaceful morning, a delicious meal).
  - Personal achievements, no matter how small.
  - Acts of kindness, both received and given.
  - The beauty in nature and surroundings.
  - Positive interactions and support from loved ones.
- Frequency: Aim for daily entries, either at the start or end of the day.
- Benefits:
  - Encourages a positive outlook by focusing on the good in life.
  - Increases mindfulness and presence in the moment.
  - Enhances emotional resilience and reduces negative emotions.
  - Strengthens relationships through appreciation of others' roles in our lives.
  - Cultivates a habit of recognizing and valuing the abundance present, even in challenging times.

Chapter 4

EMPATHETIC LISTENING

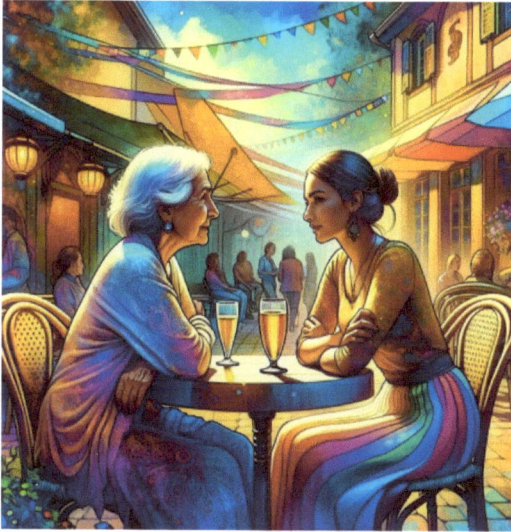

Empathetic Listening

"Empathy has no script. There is no right or wrong way to do it. It's simply listening, holding space, withholding judgment, emotionally connecting, and communicating that incredibly healing message of 'You're not alone.'" ~ **Brené Brown**

The art of empathetic listening, a fundamental skill that fosters deeper understanding, connection, and trust in our interactions with others. Unlike ordinary listening, empathetic listening requires us to fully immerse ourselves in the speaker's perspective, feeling with them and acknowledging their experience without judgment. This form of listening goes beyond merely hearing words; it involves interpreting tone, observing non-verbal cues, and offering our undivided attention and presence. By practicing empathetic listening, we not only enhance our relationships but also cultivate a compassionate and supportive environment, enabling us to connect on a more meaningful level. Empathetic listening is a powerful tool for personal and professional growth, opening the door to more genuine and fulfilling interactions.

In a world where medicine is often reduced to routine, the healing power of love and empathy can sometimes be forgotten. Yet when a patient steps into the haven of a medical facility, their hearts laden with worry and their minds clouded with anxiety, it becomes my privilege to offer more than just a clinical ear. I lend them one that hears not only their spoken worries but also their unvoiced fears. I remember well my days at an internal medicine practice, where the elderly often felt like burdens, their concerns trivialized, their presence seemingly an imposition.

One day, a very senior gentleman named Mr. Jones walked in, his devoted wife Melissa by his side, both carrying the weight of uncertainty. I listened, truly listened, giving them not just my time but my presence, and after our appointment, they expressed their gratitude for the patience and understanding I had shown. They left not just with medical advice but with a sense of being seen and heard. Their appreciation wasn't just for the care provided; it was for the empathy that was felt. They knew their well-being truly mattered to me.

To embody empathy is to extend one's heart into the practice of medicine. My patients' satisfaction sprung from the genuine concern they felt, a testament to the belief that while knowledge is vital, compassion is the true cornerstone of care. For what good is our expertise if it lacks the heartbeat of humanity? It is far greater to complement intelligence with a generous heart, and this is the rhythm to which I strive to sync every beat of my professional life.

Basics of Empathetic Listening

The basics of empathetic listening lie in distinguishing it fundamentally from the mere act of hearing. Hearing is a passive process where sound is received by the ears, but empathetic listening is an active, intentional effort to understand the speaker's message and emotions fully. This involves not just focusing on the words being said but also paying close attention to the tone of voice, facial expressions, and body language, which convey much of the emotional content.

Empathetic listening requires putting aside one's own thoughts and judgments to be fully present with the speaker, demonstrating an openness and willingness to understand their perspective. It's about listening with the heart, not just the ears, creating a space where the speaker feels seen, heard, and valued. By mastering empathetic listening, we learn to foster deeper connections and build trust, as it communicates respect and care for the speaker's experiences and feelings.

Practicing Empathy

Practicing empathy involves developing a deeper sensitivity and understanding towards the feelings and perspectives of others. This process requires us to step outside of our own experiences and enter the emotional world of another person, viewing situations and challenges through their eyes. To enhance empathy, one effective approach is to engage in active listening, where we listen to understand rather than to respond, acknowledging the other person's feelings without immediately offering advice or judgment.

Another strategy is to ask open-ended questions that encourage the speaker to express themselves more fully, thereby deepening our understanding of their experience. Visualization techniques, where we imagine ourselves in the other person's situation, can also be powerful in cultivating a genuine sense of empathy. Additionally, reflecting on our own experiences that may resonate with what others are going through can help bridge the gap of understanding. By consciously practicing these approaches, we can develop a more empathetic stance in our interactions, leading to stronger, more compassionate connections with others.

Benefits for Emotional Health

The cultivation of empathetic listening and empathy significantly benefits emotional health by paving the way for deeper and more meaningful relationships. When we actively practice empathy, we not only understand others on a more profound level but also foster an environment of trust and openness. This mutual understanding and respect facilitate stronger bonds, as individuals feel genuinely heard and valued. Empathy allows us to connect with others beyond superficial interactions, leading to relationships that are rich in emotional support and mutual compassion. Such connections provide a vital source of comfort and reassurance, contributing to our overall emotional well-being. In essence, by building empathy into our interactions, we create a foundation for relationships that nourish and sustain us, enhancing our emotional resilience and enriching our social lives.

We've navigated the profound realms of empathetic listening and empathy, uncovering their essential roles in fostering understanding, connection, and emotional health. Through practical guidance on the basics of empathetic listening and actionable strategies for practicing empathy, we've learned how these skills are pivotal in enhancing our relationships and emotional well-being. Empathy and empathetic listening are not just communication tools but bridges to deeper, more meaningful interactions, allowing us to build trust, respect, and genuine connections with others. This chapter serves as a testament to the transformative power of empathy, encouraging us to embrace and cultivate it in our daily lives for more fulfilling and compassionate relationships. As we move forward, let's carry these insights as a beacon, illuminating our path toward a more empathetic and connected world.

Take Action: Daily Active Listening

Reflective Exercise: Active Listening in Daily Conversations with Feedback Sessions

Objective: Enhance empathetic understanding and communication skills.

- **Components:**
    - **Active Listening:** Focus fully on the speaker, ignoring distractions. Pay attention not just to the words but also to non-verbal cues like tone and body language.
    - **Feedback:** After listening, provide feedback that reflects an understanding of the speaker's message and emotions. Use phrases like "What I'm hearing is..." or "It sounds like you feel..."
    - **Open-Ended Questions:** Encourage further dialogue and deeper understanding by asking questions that require more than a yes/no answer.
    - **Empathetic Responses:** Express understanding and empathy towards the speaker's situation or feelings, demonstrating genuine care and concern.
- **Practice Setting:**
    - Integrate this exercise into daily conversations with friends, family, or colleagues.
    - Schedule regular feedback sessions to discuss the experience and improve the practice.

- **Benefits:**
    - Builds stronger, more meaningful connections through improved understanding and empathy.
    - Enhances emotional intelligence by recognizing and responding to the feelings of others.
    - Develops communication skills, leading to more effective and supportive interactions.

Chapter 5

KINDNESS IN ACTION

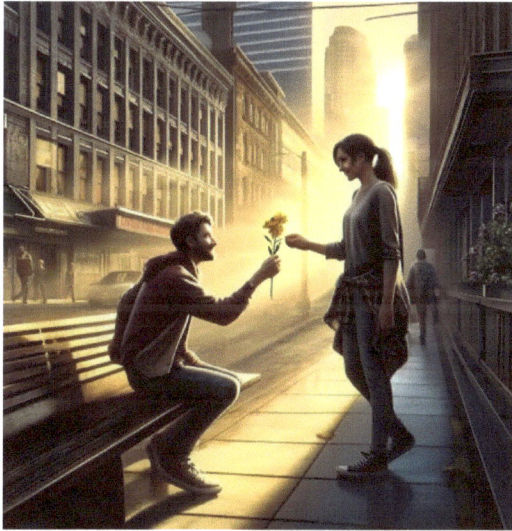

Kindness in Action

"I've learned that people will forget what you said, people will forget what you did, but people will never forget how you made them feel" ~ Maya Angelou

The vibrant world of Kindness in Action, illuminates how small acts of kindness can ripple through our lives, fostering a sense of community, enhancing well-being, and creating a more compassionate society. This exploration underscores the significance of kindness not only as a moral virtue but as a practical force for positive change. Through intentional acts of kindness, whether directed towards ourselves, others, or the environment, we engage in a powerful exchange that uplifts and connects, demonstrating the profound impact our actions can have. Kindness in Action invites us to consider how our daily choices and interactions contribute to a larger tapestry of goodwill, encouraging us to live more consciously and compassionately.

I recall working in a pediatric office as a clinical laboratory scientist, I frequently encountered children terrified at the sight of needles. This fear resonated deeply with me, having been petrified of needles myself as a child. I understood their anxiety firsthand, and I wanted to find a way to help alleviate their fears.

I put kindness into action by demonstrating bravery and normalizing the procedure. I would often volunteer to have my own blood drawn in front of the children. During these moments, I would have a coworker apply a tourniquet to my arm and proceed with the blood draw while explaining each step calmly and clearly. The goal was to show the children that while it might seem scary, it was a quick and manageable process.

This approach proved to be effective. Watching an adult calmly undergo the procedure reassured many of the children. Inspired by my example, they would then sit in the chair and bravely allow me to draw their blood. The result was remarkable: the fear in their eyes would diminish, replaced by curiosity and sometimes even pride at their own courage. Tears became rare, and the overall experience turned into a more positive one for both the children and their parents.

Through these acts of empathy and courage, we not only made the medical procedures easier for the children but also fostered an environment of trust and understanding in the office. This experience highlighted for me the profound impact of kindness and support in healthcare, particularly when addressing the fears of young patients.

Acts of Kindness

Random acts of kindness, those unexpected gestures of goodwill towards others, carry a surprisingly powerful impact on both the giver and the receiver. For the recipient, these acts can transform an ordinary day into a moment of unexpected joy, fostering feelings of gratitude and a renewed faith in the goodness of people. The emotional uplift experienced can ripple out, inspiring the receiver to pass on kindness in their own unique ways, thus creating a chain reaction of positivity. For the person performing the act, the benefits are equally profound.

Engaging in acts of kindness boosts one's own mood and sense of self-worth by fostering a connection to others and contributing to a greater cause beyond oneself. It reinforces the belief in our ability to make a difference, however small it may seem. Moreover, these acts strengthen community bonds and contribute to a culture of empathy and understanding. In essence, random acts of kindness are a testament to how simple gestures can have deep and enduring effects, nourishing a cycle of generosity and compassion in our communities.

Integrating Kindness into Daily Life

Integrating kindness into daily life begins with cultivating an awareness of the countless opportunities for kindness that each day presents. From offering a genuine compliment to a colleague or sending an encouraging message to a friend to volunteering in community service or simply being patient in stressful situations, acts of kindness can be woven into the fabric of our everyday interactions. By staying present and mindful of the needs and feelings of those around us, we can identify moments where a kind word or deed could make a significant difference. This practice not only enriches the lives of others but also enhances our own experience, fostering a sense of fulfillment and connectedness.

To make kindness a consistent part of our lives, it's helpful to set small, achievable goals for daily acts of kindness and reflect on these actions at the end of the day. Whether it's committing to smile at strangers more often, expressing gratitude regularly, or offering help without being asked, these goals can guide us in making kindness a habit. Additionally, sharing stories of kindness, whether experienced or observed, can inspire others and create a community ethos centered around compassion and support. Over time, these intentional practices not only enrich our personal well-being but also contribute to a broader culture of kindness, illustrating how each act, no matter how small, is a step towards a more compassionate world.

Benefits for Physical Health

The physiological effects of kindness on the body underscore its surprising impact on physical health, offering benefits that extend well beyond emotional well-being. Engaging in acts of kindness and experiencing kindness from others can trigger the release of the hormone oxytocin, often referred to as the "love hormone," which plays a role in lowering blood pressure and improving overall heart health. Furthermore, kindness has been linked to reduced levels of stress and anxiety, which in turn can decrease the risk of many chronic health conditions related to stress, such as heart disease and diabetes. The act of giving or receiving kindness also boosts the immune system, enhancing the body's ability to fight off infections and diseases.

Moreover, the positive emotions associated with acts of kindness can contribute to a longer, happier life. Studies have shown that people who regularly engage in kind behaviors experience less pain and discomfort, improved sleep patterns, and even longer lifespans. This is attributed to the reduction in stress hormones and the promotion of healthy lifestyle choices fostered by a positive outlook. Thus, incorporating kindness into daily life not only enriches our mental and emotional states but also offers profound benefits for our physical health, illustrating how interconnected our well-being is with how we treat ourselves and others.

We've explored the profound influence that Kindness in Action can have on our lives and the lives of those around us. Through deliberate acts of kindness, we not only enhance our own well-being and forge deeper connections with others but also contribute to a more compassionate society. This chapter has highlighted the importance of recognizing opportunities for kindness in everyday interactions and the transformative effects these gestures can have on both our physical and emotional health. By integrating kindness into our daily routines and reflecting on the impact of these actions, we cultivate a more empathetic and understanding world. As we move forward, let us carry the lessons of kindness as a guiding light, illuminating the path to a more fulfilling and connected existence.

Take Action: Intentional Acts of Kindness

Reflective Exercise: Planning and Executing a Week of Intentional Acts of Kindness

Objective: Cultivate kindness and compassion through planned, intentional acts.

- **Preparation:**
  - Identify specific acts of kindness to perform each day of the week. Consider a variety of actions, from simple gestures to more involved efforts.
  - Plan acts that are feasible and meaningful to you and that can realistically be integrated into your daily routine.
- **Daily Actions:**
  - Execute the planned act of kindness for each day. This could range from writing a thoughtful note to someone, paying a compliment, volunteering, or helping a neighbor.
  - Remain open to spontaneous opportunities for kindness in addition to the planned acts.
- **Reflection:**
  - At the end of each day, reflect on the act of kindness performed. Consider how it made you feel, the reaction of the recipient, and any changes you noticed in your interaction.
  - At the end of each week, review your experiences and reflections to assess the impact of these acts on your own well-being and on others.

- **Benefits:**
    - Enhances personal and communal well-being.
    - Fosters a positive mood and outlook.
    - Encourages the development of a habit of kindness.
    - Strengthens connections with others and builds community.

Chapter 6

NURTURING RELATIONSHIPS

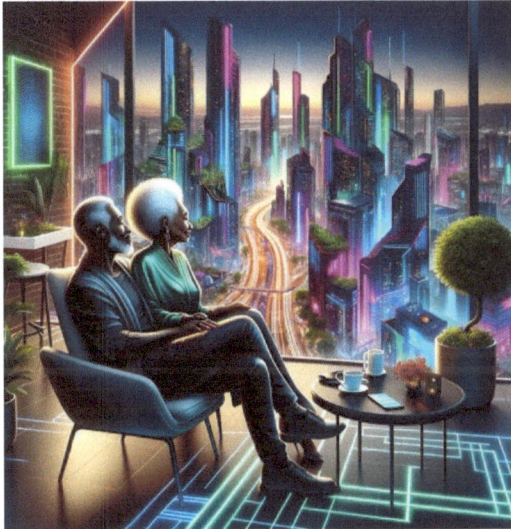

Nurturing Relationships

Nurturing Relationships is an art, a crucial aspect of leading a fulfilled and balanced life. It explores the importance of cultivating deep, meaningful connections with others, whether they be familial ties, friendships, or romantic partnerships. This chapter offers insights into the foundational elements that sustain and enrich relationships, such as effective communication, empathy, mutual respect, and shared experiences. By understanding and applying these principles, we learn not only to maintain but also to nurture and strengthen the bonds that tie us to one another. Nurturing relationships requires intentional effort and understanding, but the rewards—a support network filled with love, understanding, and connection—far outweigh the investment, enriching our lives in profound ways.

I was intentional about staying connected with my paternal grandparents. Especially with my grandmother. My relationship with my grannie was always anchored by a deep sense of respect and affection, shaped significantly by our shared love for communication and medicine. Growing up, I was captivated by stories of her life as a registered nurse, which she often shared. These stories not only bridged our generational gap but also strengthened our bond in profound ways.

When I pursued my academic career, which took me to institutions far from home, visiting my grannie became increasingly challenging. However, the physical distance only deepened our commitment to maintaining and nurturing our relationship. We chose a rather non-traditional yet deeply personal method of communication: writing letters.

Our exchange of letters began as a simple means of updating each other on our lives but soon evolved into a cherished ritual. I would send handwritten letters from various corners of the country detailing my life and academic experiences. Each letter I penned was a meditation on my daily life, filled with challenges and triumphs, written in the hope of bringing her closer to my world.

In return, my grannie filled her letters with tales and insights from her days as a nurse. Her descriptions were vivid and educational, providing a window into a past era of medical practice and allowing me to see the parallels and differences in our professional journeys. This exchange was not just about staying informed about each other's lives; it was a unique opportunity to learn from her experiences and wisdom.

The beauty of our letter writing was its simplicity and the anticipation it built. Each letter was a tangible expression of love and care, something physical that could be held, cherished, and revisited. The waiting made the connection feel even more special because it taught patience and the excitement of receiving something so personal in the mail was always a highlight of my week.

Moreover, this ongoing dialogue created an archival narrative of our lives, a testament to our evolving relationship and changing worlds. It was a way to document our growth and learning, preserved in ink and paper. Through her letters, I gained not just personal advice but also a historical perspective on the medical field, enriching my own educational journey and providing a foundation upon which I could build my future.

This tradition of letter writing has taught me the importance of nurturing relationships through consistent, thoughtful communication. It has shown me that strong bonds are maintained not through proximity but through the willingness to share and listen, to teach and learn. Our letters have become a cherished inheritance, a meaningful legacy of a relationship that transcended time and distance through the simple, powerful act of writing.

It's my hope that others find unique ways to connect with their loved ones, especially across distances. Whether through letters, calls, or the more modern form of communication, the essence lies in the effort to stay connected and the mutual exchange of knowledge and affection, which are the hallmarks of any nurturing relationship.

The Importance of Relationships

The significance of relationships in influencing our mental and physical health cannot be overstated. On a psychological level, strong, supportive relationships provide a sense of belonging and purpose, significantly reducing feelings of loneliness and isolation. They act as a buffer against stress, anxiety, and depression, with positive interactions boosting self-esteem and overall happiness. The emotional support derived from close connections enables individuals to navigate life's challenges with greater resilience, contributing to a healthier mental state. Relationships encourage personal growth and understanding, fostering an environment where individuals can thrive emotionally and mentally.

Physically, the benefits of healthy relationships are equally compelling. Studies have shown that individuals with robust social support systems have a lower risk of numerous health problems, including cardiovascular disease, high blood pressure, and weakened immune systems. Positive interpersonal connections can even influence longevity, with research suggesting that strong social bonds are associated with a reduced risk of premature death. The stress-reducing effects of good relationships also play a critical role in physical well-being, as chronic stress is a known risk factor for a variety of health issues. Thus, nurturing relationships not only enriches our emotional lives but also has a tangible impact on our physical health, underscoring the interconnectedness of social connections and overall well-being.

Building and Maintaining Strong Bonds

Building and maintaining strong bonds in any relationship hinges on the pillars of effective communication, trust, and mutual support. Effective communication goes beyond mere exchange of information; it's about sharing thoughts, feelings, and needs in a way that is clear, open, and receptive. It involves active listening, empathy, and the willingness to understand the other person's perspective. This open line of communication fosters trust, an essential element in any relationship. Trust is built over time through consistency, reliability, and integrity, creating a safe space for vulnerability and genuine connection. It's the foundation that allows relationships to withstand challenges and grow stronger over time.

Mutual support, the third pillar, involves offering encouragement, assistance, and understanding to one another, celebrating successes, and being there through difficulties. It's about being responsive to each other's needs and making an effort to contribute positively to the other person's life. This support strengthens the bond between individuals, reinforcing the sense of a shared journey and mutual growth. Together, effective communication, trust, and mutual support create a robust framework for building and maintaining relationships that are not only enduring but also enriching, allowing individuals to navigate life's ups and downs with confidence and companionship.

Benefits of Compassionate Conflict Resolution

Compassionate conflict resolution is a vital skill in nurturing and maintaining healthy relationships, emphasizing the approach to disagreements with empathy and understanding. This method involves recognizing the validity of the other person's feelings and perspective, even when they differ from one's own. By prioritizing the relationship over the need to be right, individuals can navigate conflicts in a way that strengthens rather than weakens bonds. Compassionate conflict resolution encourages open communication, where both parties feel heard and respected. It involves actively listening to the other person's concerns, expressing your own in a non-confrontational way, and collaboratively seeking solutions that address both parties' needs. This approach fosters a safe environment for addressing issues, reducing the likelihood of resentment and promoting mutual understanding.

Implementing empathy in conflict resolution means striving to see the situation from the other person's viewpoint and acknowledging their emotions. This empathetic stance helps in de-escalating tension and facilitates a more constructive dialogue. It's about finding common ground and working together towards a resolution that benefits both parties, reflecting a deep respect for the relationship. By adopting a compassionate approach to resolving disagreements, individuals can transform potential conflicts into opportunities for growth and deeper connection. This not only resolves the immediate issue but also builds a framework for handling future challenges in a healthy, constructive manner, reinforcing the resilience and depth of the relationship.

We've journeyed through the essential terrain of nurturing relationships, uncovering the profound ways in which our connections with others influence our mental and physical health and the foundational elements required to build and maintain strong, meaningful bonds. We've delved into the importance of effective communication, trust, mutual support, and compassionate conflict resolution, highlighting how these components are integral to deepening our relationships. The chapter emphasized that nurturing relationships is a dynamic, ongoing process that enriches our lives, providing a sense of belonging, support, and joy. Through intentional actions and reflective exercises, we've seen how we can assess and enhance our most valued connections, making them even more rewarding. As we move forward, let us carry the insights and practices from this chapter into our daily lives, continually striving to nurture the relationships that form the heart of our shared human experience.

Take Action: Leveling Up Valued Relationships

Reflective Exercise: Assessing and Deepening One's Most Valued Relationships

- **Steps:**
    - Identification: Start by identifying the relationships you value most, considering family, friends, and significant others.
    - Assessment: Reflect on the current state of these relationships. Consider aspects such as communication, trust, support, and satisfaction.
    - Recognition: Acknowledge areas of strength and areas needing improvement within each relationship.
    - Goal Setting: For each relationship, set specific goals aimed at deepening the connection. Goals may include improving communication, spending more quality time together, or addressing unresolved conflicts.
    - Action Plans: Develop actionable steps to achieve these goals. This could involve scheduling regular check-ins, planning shared activities, or learning more about compassionate conflict resolution.
    - Implementation: Begin to put your action plans into practice, keeping your goals in mind during interactions.
    - Reflection: Regularly reflect on the progress made towards your goals, and adjust your actions as necessary to continue nurturing and deepening these important bonds.
- **Benefits:**
    - Enhances mutual understanding and empathy within valued relationships.
    - Strengthens emotional bonds and increases overall relationship satisfaction.
    - Fosters a supportive and nurturing environment for personal and mutual growth.

Dr. Tinille T. Jenkins, DMS, PA-C, MSMS, CLS (ASCP)

Chapter 7

HOLISTIC SELF-CARE

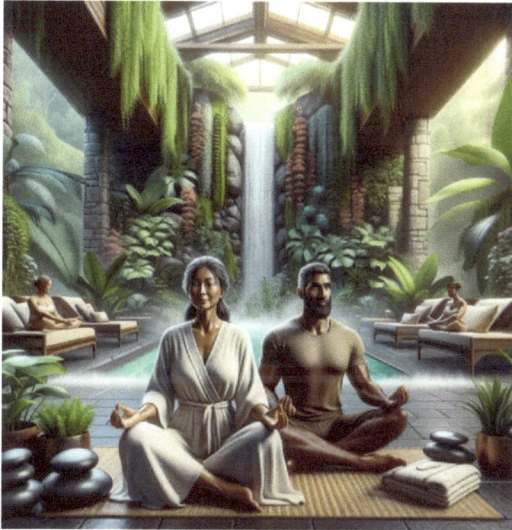

Holistic Self-Care

Shifting our focus towards Holistic Self-Care, an essential practice that emphasizes the nourishment of mind, body, and spirit in unison. This approach to self-care transcends mere physical wellness, advocating for a comprehensive strategy that fosters emotional resilience, mental clarity, and spiritual fulfillment. By exploring the interconnectedness of these aspects of our being, the chapter guides us through various practices and philosophies aimed at achieving a balanced and enriched life. Holistic self-care is presented not just as an act of personal health but as a profound journey of self-discovery and transformation, inviting us to engage deeply with our inner selves and the world around us, thereby cultivating a life of wellness, harmony, and purpose.

Let me share a personal slice of my daily life, one that became a cornerstone of my holistic self-care practice. Every morning, as I drove to school, my car transformed into more than just a vehicle; it became a vessel of learning and growth. The serene early hours offer a perfect backdrop as Catherine Ponder's inspirational words flow through the speakers from my Audible account. Her guidance doesn't just fill the space; it permeates my being, encouraging me to dream beyond my current circumstances and visualize the success I am destined to achieve.

My routine didn't end with the drive. Each day begins purposefully with prayer and meditation in the quiet comfort of my apartment, where I connect deeply with myself before the world wakes. Here, surrounded by the soft dawn light, I focus on my breath and the aspirations that shape my path forward: my faith. The prayer and meditation set the tone for the day, grounding me in peace and clarity. Afterward, I affirm my worth and capabilities by reading aloud positive affirmations, each word reinforcing the foundation of my self-belief and fortitude.

This structured regimen of physical, mental, and emotional care formed the backbone of my journey toward personal fulfillment and professional success. These practices arm me against life's challenges, fostering resilience and joy in my pursuit of a future where my then struggles were merely echoes of ugliness that would soon be defeated. These rituals, inspired me and had transformative powers of integrating holistic self-care into my life. Try them!

.

Compassionate Self-Care

Compassionate Self-Care frames the practice of taking care of oneself not just as a routine necessity but as a profound act of self-respect and kindness. This perspective encourages us to approach self-care with the same empathy and consideration we would offer to a loved one, recognizing that nurturing our well-being is fundamental to our capacity to thrive and support others. By viewing self-care through this lens, we shift from seeing it as a selfish indulgence to understanding it as a vital component of a healthy, balanced life. Compassionate self-care involves listening attentively to our own needs, whether they be physical rest, emotional support, or mental relaxation, and responding with actions that reflect a deep care for our well-being.

Adopting this approach also means forgiving ourselves for not always meeting external expectations and acknowledging that taking time for self-care is a necessary step in maintaining our health and happiness. It allows us to set healthy boundaries, prioritize our needs, and make choices that align with our well-being, reinforcing the idea that self-care is a rightful act of self-love. Compassionate Self-Care encourages a gentle, understanding attitude toward ourselves, especially in moments of stress or challenge, promoting a holistic approach to health that integrates the needs of the mind, body, and spirit. Through this practice, we learn to cherish ourselves with kindness, paving the way for a more fulfilling and compassionate life journey.

Physical, Mental, and Emotional Self-Care

Integrating compassionate practices into all aspects of self-care, physical, mental, and emotional ensures a holistic approach to well-being that honors the interconnectedness of our human experience. Physical self-care goes beyond exercise and nutrition; it's about treating the body with kindness, recognizing its signals of stress or fatigue, and responding with nurturing actions, like rest or movement that feels joyous rather than obligatory. Mental self-care involves engaging in activities that stimulate and rest the mind in equal measure, be it through meditation, reading, or creative pursuits, allowing for growth and recovery. Emotionally, compassionate self-care means allowing ourselves to feel and express a wide range of emotions without judgment, seeking support when needed, and practicing self-forgiveness and positivity.

By weaving compassionate practices into these three pillars of self-care, we create a self-care routine that is responsive and adaptive to our changing needs, promoting overall health and happiness. This approach encourages us to be mindful of our self-talk and the choices we make in caring for ourselves, ensuring they come from a place of love and respect. It's about recognizing that self-care is a personal journey, one that is unique to each individual and that the most effective practices are those that resonate with our own values and circumstances. Through this integrative and compassionate approach, we foster a deeper connection with ourselves, enhancing our resilience, contentment, and the quality of our engagement with life.

Benefits of a Personalized Self-Care Routine

Developing a personalized self-care routine that nurtures the whole self requires a mindful approach to understanding what truly benefits and rejuvenates you physically, mentally, and emotionally. Begin by reflecting on activities that bring you joy, relaxation, and a sense of fulfillment. Consider incorporating practices that address all aspects of your well-being, such as physical exercise that you enjoy, mindfulness or meditation for mental clarity, creative hobbies for emotional expression, and social activities that foster connection. It's important to listen to your body and mind, adjusting your self-care practices as your needs and circumstances change. Remember, flexibility is key; what works for you one day may not work the next, and that's okay.

When crafting your routine, aim for balance rather than perfection. Start small, with one or two practices, and gradually build your routine to prevent overwhelm. Schedule these activities into your day as non-negotiable appointments with yourself, ensuring they are prioritized. However, remain open to modifying your routine as you discover what best supports your well-being. Incorporating variety can keep your routine fresh and engaging, encouraging you to maintain these beneficial practices long-term. Ultimately, a personalized self-care routine is about making a commitment to yourself and recognizing that caring for your well-being is not a luxury but a necessity for a healthy, balanced life.

We've embraced the concept of Holistic Self-Care, recognizing it as a multifaceted practice that nourishes mind, body, and spirit. Through compassionate self-care, integrating practices into all aspects of our well-being, and crafting personalized routines, we've uncovered strategies to support our overall health in a comprehensive, meaningful way. This chapter highlighted the importance of viewing self-care as an essential, ongoing journey of self-respect and kindness. As we move forward, let these insights inspire us to cultivate a self-care practice that reflects our unique needs and fosters a deep, enduring sense of wellness. Embracing holistic self-care empowers us to lead more balanced, fulfilled lives, demonstrating that the greatest kindness we can offer ourselves is the commitment to our own well-being.

As we reach the conclusion of our journey through the pages of this book, we've explored a tapestry of practices and philosophies centered on wellness, mindful awareness, self-compassion, gratitude, empathetic listening, nurturing relationships, and holistic self-care. Each chapter has been a step toward understanding how these interconnected elements contribute to a life lived with intention, kindness, and balance. We've probed into the importance of being present, embracing ourselves with compassion, cherishing our connections with others, and nurturing our entire being with thoughtful self-care.

Take Action: Design A Self-Care Plan

Reflective Exercise: Designing a Self-Care Plan with Compassionate Habits at Its Core

Objective: Create a personalized self-care routine that prioritizes compassion and well-being.

- **Steps:**

  - Self-Assessment: Begin by evaluating your current physical, mental, and emotional needs. Identify areas that require more attention or improvement.

  - Goal Setting: Define clear, attainable goals for each aspect of your well-being. Ensure these goals reflect a compassionate approach to self-care.

  - Activity Selection: Choose activities that align with your goals and bring you joy. Include practices for physical health (e.g., yoga, walking), mental clarity (e.g., meditation, journaling), and emotional well-being (e.g., creative hobbies, therapy).

  - Plan Integration: Schedule these activities into your daily or weekly routine, treating them as essential appointments with yourself.

  - Flexibility: Remain open to adjusting your plan as needed. Recognize that your self-care needs may change over time, and allow your routine to evolve accordingly.

- **Reflection and Adjustment:**

    o Regularly reflect on the effectiveness of your self-care plan. Consider what's working well and what might need tweaking.

    o Make adjustments based on your reflections to ensure your self-care routine continues to meet your needs effectively.

- **Benefits:**

    o Enhances overall well-being by addressing the needs of the mind, body, and spirit.

    o Promotes a positive and compassionate relationship with oneself.

    o Increases resilience, happiness, and fulfillment by nurturing all aspects of personal health.

Compassion Assessment

Below, rate yourself on a scale from 1-5 on how accurate the statements are – 1 means "not accurate at all" and 5 means "most accurate."

Once you've rated yourself for each statement, total up your scores and then use the Answer Key to determine your next steps.

Compassion Assessment	Self-Rating
I genuinely like being kind to others	
I often find myself feeling empathy for both friends and strangers.	
I make a conscious effort to help others without expecting anything in return.	
I am sensitive to the feelings of people around me.	
I often take the time to listen to someone else's problem, even if I am busy.	
I regularly perform small acts of kindness for others.	
I feel a sense of purpose when I am able to alleviate someone else's suffering.	
I am non-judgmental.	
I find it easy to put myself in another person's shoes and see things from their perspective.	
I am patient with others, even when they make mistakes.	
I often notice when someone needs emotional support.	
I make an effort to include everyone when in a group setting, ensuring no one feels left out.	
I am quick to offer assistance to someone who appears to be in distress.	
I actively listen to others, showing genuine interest in understanding their experiences.	

I regularly express gratitude towards others for the big and small things they do.	
I am mindful of my words and actions, especially how they affect others.	
I forgive others easily and prefer to focus on positive outcomes.	
I dedicate part of my time to volunteer activities or community service.	
I am often moved to act when I hear about injustices or suffering in the world.	
I strive to be an advocate for those who are less fortunate or unable to speak for themselves.	
Total Score	

Compassionate people are the heart of their communities, instinctively empathizing with others and acting to alleviate distress wherever they see it. They genuinely seek to understand others' feelings, offering support through both small acts of kindness and significant gestures. These individuals recognize our deep interconnectedness and strive to uplift everyone around them, finding deep fulfillment in enriching others' lives.

Score 0-65

The Fundamentals of Compassion are Missing

The bad news is that your compassion qualities are missing core fundamentals. This is likely not a surprise to you.

However, the good news is that you can grow and improve on your core qualities. Get some coaching to expedite the process.

Read this book with an open mind and make notes of 1 or 2 areas that you can excel in and study to master. You may have to review the chapters you have already completed. Next, intentionally mentor someone else to practice compassion along with you. Having an accountability partner is helpful.

> Score 66-78
>
> Compassionate at Heart and Growing

If your score landed you here, you are on track to becoming the Compassionate person others will admire.

Be intentional about making a conscious effort to shift your behaviors to be more in line with a true Compassionate Seeker. Leveling up your efforts in one or two areas will propel you to the top rank. Support can be helpful to expedite success. Try coaching.

> Score 79-100
>
> Compassion Seeker

Since your score landed you here, it is safe to say that you are a compassionate person. This should excite you!

For you, the biggest compassionate hurdle to overcome is…

_____. I would like some assistance in working through "it." Contact Coach Tina FJ: Connect@drtinafj.com

About The Author

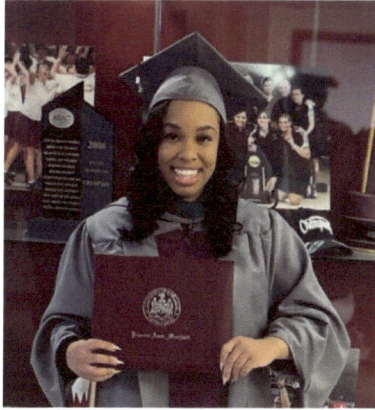

Dr. Tinille Tina Jenkins, DMS, PA-C, MSMS, CLS (ASCP), finished her undergraduate at Winston Salem University in Winston Salem, NC, in 2010 with a degree in Clinical Laboratory Science, and soon after she became a Board-Certified Clinical Laboratory Scientist. She received her first Masters in Medical Science from Ponce Health Sciences University, and her second Masters in Medical Science, Physician Associate from the University of Maryland Eastern Shore. Lastly, Tinille received her doctorate from Butler University.

Tinille absolutely loves almost anything medical. She is an author and a loving and compassionate person. In fact, she is a Compassion Seeker (*check out the Compassion Assessment*). Tinille enjoys homemade chocolate chip cookies and Maryland crabs. She makes her home in Bowie, Maryland, with her parents and her younger sister.

Chapter 8

BONUS CHAPTER: THE 360°
HEALTH CARE: PREVENTION TO
PROTECTION TO PRESERVATION

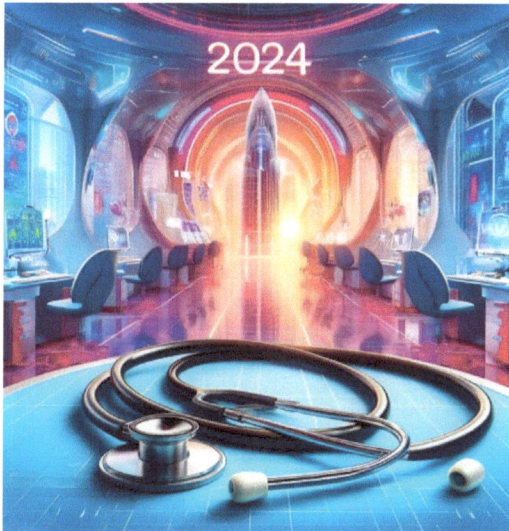

The 360° Health Care Plan: From Prevention To Protection To Preservation

"The eye is the lamp of the body. If your eyes are healthy, your whole body will be full of light. But if your eyes are unhealthy, your whole body will be full of darkness."
~ Matthew 6:22-24 NKJ

Welcome to *The 360° Health Care: From Prevention to Protection to Preservation.* This is a comprehensive look at the core pillars of health care that support our quality of life. In this chapter, we'll explore general health, eye care, and skin care, three vital areas that create a well-rounded approach to feeling and looking our best together. From the essentials of annual check-ups and lab work that help us stay ahead of potential issues to the protective steps we can take for our eyes and skin, we'll look into how each of these areas contributes to our overall well-being. Whether it's the preventive steps that keep us in balance, the protective habits that shield us from harm, or the daily practices that preserve our health for the long haul, this chapter will help you make sense of your visits and give you practical tools to take charge of your health journey.

Healthcare Protection, Prevention, and Preservation

Caring for our health, especially through primary care and internal medicine, is like nurturing the foundation of a sturdy, time-honored home. It is all about creating a secure and resilient structure for the years ahead. Regular visits to a primary care physician are not just routine; they're a proactive step toward maintaining balance in our bodies, catching early warning signs, and setting the stage for a healthier future. During these visits, healthcare providers focus on crucial health measurements that help to track our overall wellness and detect issues early.

While I was in clinical rotations, I encountered a seasoned woman devoted to her health and wellness. Her dedication to attending annual check-ups as part of her commitment to preventative care exemplified her proactive approach to maintaining her well-being. During what she believed would be a routine visit, her provider noticed irregularities during an exam, prompting an in-office ECG. The results revealed ST elevations, a critical finding suggestive of an acute myocardial infarction (heart attack). Recognizing the urgency of the situation, the provider immediately called an ambulance, and she was swiftly transported to the hospital for life-saving treatment. Her commitment to regular check-ups and preventative care ultimately saved her life, highlighting the importance of proactive health measures.

Every adult, from 18 years and beyond, can benefit from having their essential health markers checked at each visit. These health markers usually include blood pressure measurements, heart rate, weight, and temperature.

- Blood Pressure: Ideal blood pressure for most adults should be below 120/80 mmHg. Readings consistently above 130/80 mmHg indicate high blood pressure or hypertension, which raises the risk for heart disease and stroke.

- Heart Rate: A regular resting heart rate for adults ranges from 60 to 100 beats per minute. Regularly low or high readings can signal underlying issues needing further investigation.

- Weight: While weight itself varies considerably, tracking it helps in assessing changes that could signal health concerns, especially in relation to Body Mass Index (BMI), which ideally falls between 18.5 and 24.9.

- Temperature: Normal body temperature typically ranges between 97°F and 99°F. Any variation outside this range may indicate infection, inflammation, or other health concerns.

Beyond these measurements, a thorough health check-up often includes lab tests that offer insights into our body's inner workings:

- Complete Metabolic Panel (CMP): This test checks kidney and liver function, electrolytes, and blood glucose levels.
    - Glucose: Normal fasting glucose levels range from 70 to 99 mg/dL. Levels of 100-125 mg/dL indicate prediabetes, and above 126 mg/dL on two separate tests can signal diabetes.

o Creatinine and Blood Urea Nitrogen (BUN) are checked to assess kidney health, with creatinine levels typically ranging between 0.6 and 1.2 mg/dL and BUN from 7 to 20 mg/dL.

o Electrolytes like sodium (135-145 mmol/L), potassium (3.6-5.2 mmol/L), and calcium (8.5-10.2 mg/dL) help gauge hydration and overall balance.

- Complete Blood Count (CBC): A CBC measures red and white blood cells and platelets, which can indicate conditions like anemia, infection, bone marrow disorders, autoimmune diseases, inflammation and hematological disorders.

    o Red Blood Cells (RBCs): Typical values for men are 4.7-6.1 10^6 cell/μL, and for women, 4.2-5.4 10^6 cell/μL.

    $\Rightarrow$ Hemoglobin: Should be between 13.8 and 17.2 g/dL for men and 12.1 to 15.1 g/dL for women.

    o White Blood Cells (WBCs): A normal range is 4,500 to 11,000 cells per microliter, while elevated levels can indicate infection.

    o Platelet reference range is 150,000–450,000/μL.

- Lipid Panel: This test includes cholesterol and triglycerides, which are essential for heart health.

    o Total Cholesterol: Below 200 mg/dL is desirable.

- LDL (bad cholesterol): Should be less than 100mg/dL; above 160 mg/dL is high.

- HDL (good cholesterol): Above 60 mg/dL is considered protective.

- Triglycerides: Should be below 150 mg/dL, with higher levels raising heart disease risk.

- Hemoglobin A1c: For a look at long-term blood sugar levels, a hemoglobin A1c test is done.

- A1c levels below 5.7% are standard, while levels between 5.7% and 6.4% indicate prediabetes, and 6.5% or higher on two separate tests confirm diabetes.

In addition to standard checks, certain screenings are essential for comprehensive adult care:

- Bone Density Test (DEXA): Recommended for women over 65 and men over 70, this scan assesses bone strength and identifies early osteoporosis risk, especially useful for those with family history or long-term steroid use.

- Pulmonary Function Test (PFT): Measures lung capacity and airflow to detect respiratory issues like asthma or COPD, particularly valuable for those with respiratory symptoms or high exposure to pollutants.

- Low-Dose Computed Tomography (LDCT): For adults 50+ with significant smoking history, an LDCT scan detects early lung cancer signs more effectively than standard X-rays.

- Electrocardiogram (ECG): Records heart activity to identify irregular rhythms or cardiovascular issues, advised for those with a family history of heart disease, hypertension, or diabetes care.

Think of each health check-up as a pit stop on your life's journey. It is a chance to refuel, fine-tune, and make sure everything's running smoothly for the miles ahead. From blood pressure to bone density, these routine checks give us the inside scoop on how our bodies are holding up, often catching issues before they become roadblocks. While it may seem like a lot to keep track of, each test is a small investment toward a healthier, longer life. So, next time you're at the doctor's office, remember: these visits are more than just boxes to check, they're the proactive steps that keep you strong, resilient, and ready for the road ahead!

Take Action: Schedule your Primary Care Exams

YEAR	DATE	TIME	DOCTOR

Take Action: Schedule your Specialty Care Exams

(i.e., Xrays, MRIs, Cardiology, Orthopedic, Gynocology, etc.)

YEAR	DATE	TIME	DOCTOR

Eye Care Health

Windows through which we perceive the world… our eyes. It's not just about seeing well today; it's about ensuring that we continue to witness life's beauty well into the future. This section is your companion on a path to comprehensive eye care, encompassing everything from the essentials of regular check-ups to the subtleties of dietary choices that can fortify your vision. As we delve into the pages, we'll explore how to guard against the unseen dangers of ultraviolet rays, the impacts of screens on our delicate sight, and the simple steps we can take to maintain ocular health.

Consider this section a mosaic, where each piece is a screening, a sunglass, a diet rich in leafy greens, or the conscious effort to rest our eyes from the digital glow, and they all come together to form a complete picture of eye wellness. Here, you'll find not just guidelines but a philosophy that integrates eye health into the very fabric of a well-lived life. So, let's embark on this visionary quest, where each stride we take is a step toward clarity, comfort, and, ultimately, a deeper appreciation of the world around us through eyes that are cared for and cherished.

Before we get started, I want to share my eye story, which started when I was pretty young. My childhood was shadowed by a case of mistaken identity; I was given glasses for a sight issue that was never really there. It wasn't my eyes that had trouble, but my brain's way of piecing together the puzzles of letters and words. It is a little something called dyslexia. Those glasses? I'd ditch them at any chance I got, a small act of rebellion against a solution that was never meant for me.

The real breakthrough came with the correct diagnosis. Imagine a light switch that hesitates for a moment before flooding a room with light. That is how my mind works. Spatial dyslexia is my specific travel partner, causing a lag in the connection between seeing words and processing their meaning. I learned to exist in this brief silence before comprehension, to 'wait for it' as understanding leisurely made its way through the corridors of my cognition. Another analogy for Spatial dyslexia is that I lived in a brief echo of time, waiting for the words to make sense. This wasn't an ailment to cure but a reality to embrace, a different rhythm to learn, and I did.

Now, I see clearly in more ways than one. My vision is a sharp 20/15, and I navigate the world with the understanding that dyslexia, in its tangled web, is not just a challenge but a gift. It lets me see the layers of life with a richness other might miss. And in a twist of fate, I worked in an ophthalmology office. I was able to be a guardian of the very sense I once struggled to understand. It's a role that celebrates the full circle of my journey: from those discarded glasses to a position built on the beauty of sight, both given and perceived.

Prevent Eye Problems

Taking care of our eyes is a bit like looking after a precious family heirloom; it requires attention, care, and a proactive approach. The simple act of scheduling regular eye exams isn't just another to-do on our list; it's a commitment to safeguarding our most cherished sense, our sight. These screenings are like secret sentinels, silently scouting for trouble before it becomes a more significant battle. They're especially vital for our little ones, who have so much to see and learn, and for those of us who've watched the seasons change more than a few times or for anyone with a health condition that could cast a shadow over their vision.

Now, let's talk about those stealthy health issues that like to lurk in the background, such as diabetes and high blood pressure. They're like the quiet culprits that, without a watchful eye, might sneak up on our sight. Managing these conditions isn't just about taking pills or following a diet; it's about being the guardian of our own vision. By keeping these conditions in check, we're not just avoiding eye problems; we're ensuring that every sunrise, every smiling face, and every autumn leaf remains crisp, clear, and full of color. After all, our eyes are the storytellers of our lives, and we want them to tell a tale as vivid and as full of life as the world around us.

Protect Your Eyes

When it comes to the guardians of your body, your eyes are on the frontline, and they deserve armor befitting their role.

Whether you're diving into a home improvement project, playing a weekend game of hoops, or chipping away in your workshop, think of protective eyewear as your personal shield. Safety glasses, goggles, and eye guards are the unsung heroes, the quiet defenders against the unpredictable. They're not just accessories; they're essential gear in your daily quest to keep your eyes safe from life's little skirmishes.

But protection isn't only about what you can see; it's also about the invisible rays that the sun sends cascading down on us. Just as you wouldn't step into a bright day without sunscreen, don't overlook your eyes when it comes to UV protection. A good pair of sunglasses does more than add mystique to your look. They are a barrier against the UV rays that can lead to cataracts and a suite of other eye concerns. When choosing these trusty companions, look for ones that promise to block out 99% of UV-A and UV-B radiation, and consider it an investment in a clearer, brighter future.

In this digital era, our eyes are glued to screens more often than not, and it's easy to forget that they weren't designed for a world reduced to pixels and LEDs. Embrace the 20-20-20 rule as a rhythmic dance for your eyes: every 20 minutes, entice them to gaze upon something 20 feet away for at least 20 seconds. This small practice is like a gentle massage for your eye muscles, a brief vacation on your busy day. And while you're at it, fine-tune your screens with the correct brightness, wear an anti-glare guard, or slip on a pair of computer glasses to filter out the harshness. Think of these steps as little acts of kindness, tiny love letters to your hardworking eyes.

Preserve Eye Care

Nourishing your body is like tending to a garden; what you put into the soil determines the health of everything that grows from it. When it comes to your eyes, the bounty you need comes from a banquet of omega-3 fatty acids, lutein, zinc, and vitamins C and E nutrients that are like secret agents warding off age-related eye diseases. Picture each leafy green, each piece of salmon, and each nut as a gift to your eyes, a kind of health insurance that's as delicious as it is wise. Eating well is like giving your eyes a suit of armor against the ravages of time, a way to keep seeing the world in all its splendor.

Then there's smoking, a dragon that wreaks havoc on more than just your lungs. Its smoky tendrils can obscure the clarity of your vision, leading to cataracts and macular degeneration. But here's the good news: slaying this dragon and casting away the cigarettes can be like lifting a veil from your eyes, protecting those delicate windows to your soul. And while you're in the business of safeguarding your sight, remember that maintaining a healthy weight isn't just about fitting into your favorite jeans. It is about staying light on your feet so that diseases that cloud your vision can't catch you.

As for eye care, it's a family affair. Educating yourself and your loved ones about the signs of eye problems is like learning the language of your body, understanding what it needs and when it needs help. Keep a lookout for red eyes, the squint of strain, or the haze of changing vision; these are whispers from your body, cues that it's time to act. And don't forget to keep your eyewear current; glasses and contacts are your allies, and they need to be in top shape to fight alongside you. Lastly, embrace vigilance. Any change in your vision is a signal, perhaps a call to arms, and it pays to heed it swiftly. In the realm of eye health, being alert and ready to act is the mark of a true guardian.

As we draw the curtains on this subject, let's hold onto the simple yet powerful truth we've uncovered: our eyes are invaluable treasures that demand our respect and care. Embracing a lifestyle that cherishes eye health goes beyond mere maintenance. It's an act of profound self-respect. The steps we've journeyed through together, from nurturing our bodies with nutrients to shielding our eyes from the sun's glare, are rituals of protection for our vision. Giving up smoking, staying vigilant about our weight, and educating ourselves are all pledges we make not just to our eyes but to our continued experience of the world's beauty.

Remember, each choice we make, each habit we foster, is a brushstroke in the masterpiece of our well-being. The practices we've explored are not just acts of care but acts of love but love for the moments we capture with our eyes, the memories we paint in vibrant colors, and the future vistas we yearn to see. Let's step forward from this chapter with a renewed commitment to this art of seeing, carrying with us the wisdom to preserve, protect, and prioritize the health of our eyes. Our eyes are the very lenses through which we behold the tapestry of life.

Take Action: Schedule your Eye Care Exams

YEAR	DATE	TIME	DOCTOR

Hair, Nail, and Skin Care

Here's your guide to the essentials of hair, nail, and skin care. It is a bit of daily magic that goes beyond just looking good! This section looks into the hidden side of beauty care, showing you how a few smart choices can keep your skin glowing, hair strong, and nails smooth and resilient. Think of it as a backstage pass to preventing the common issues that pop up over time, whether it's through skin cancer screenings to catch anything suspicious early or allergy tests to make sure that new lotion won't cause a surprise breakout. From nutritional check-ups to keep your skin and hair well-nourished to hormone tests that clue you into what's going on under the surface, this is where prevention meets self-care in the most practical (and rewarding) way. So, get ready to learn a few tricks of the trade that can keep your skin, hair, and nails healthy for the long haul. Why? Because feeling good on the inside and out never goes out of style!

Hair, Nail, and Skin Care Prevention

Preventing issues with skin, hair, and nails goes beyond daily routines; it also involves strategic testing to catch underlying health factors early. Regular skin cancer screenings by a dermatologist can detect early signs of cancer, particularly for those at higher risk, such as individuals with a family history or high sun exposure. Allergy testing through patch tests identifies product sensitivities, preventing allergic reactions that can impact skin and scalp health. Additionally, nutritional blood tests for vitamins and minerals reveal deficiencies that can lead to brittle nails, hair loss, and skin dryness. Hormonal testing checks for imbalances affecting hair growth, skin texture, and nail strength, while genetic testing can uncover predispositions to skin conditions like psoriasis, guiding preventative strategies.

For persistent or unusual skin lesions, a biopsy may be recommended to rule out cancer, providing crucial early detection. Dermatologists can also perform hair and scalp analyses to monitor for signs of damage and prevent conditions like alopecia or dermatitis. Cortisol testing measures stress-related hormone levels, which can affect skin, hair, and nail health, allowing for tailored stress management approaches. Norepinephrine testing assesses chronic stress impacts, such as accelerated hair graying and skin sensitivity, and oxidative stress testing measures biomarkers that signal potential skin aging and damage from free radicals, supporting antioxidant intervention.

Hair, Nail, and Skin Care Protection

When it comes to safeguarding your appearance, think of your skin, hair, and nails as frontline defenders, and treat them to the care they deserve. Whether you're braving the sun on a hike, styling hair for a big event, or handling chemicals during a DIY project, consider your protective measures as essential armor.

Sunscreen, gloves, and hats are your quiet guardians, shielding your skin, hair, and nails from the daily skirmishes of life. These aren't just accessories but vital tools in maintaining health and vitality.

Protection isn't only about the obvious, like sun exposure; it's also about the invisible effects of UV rays, pollution, and environmental stressors. Just as you'd protect your face with sunscreen, don't forget to shield your hair with UV sprays and your nails with nourishing oils. Opt for a broad-spectrum sunscreen for your skin, offering at least SPF 30 to defend against both UVA and UVB rays, and invest in products that keep your hair and nails resilient under the sun. These simple additions to your routine do more than protect; they preserve the health and vibrancy of your natural look.

Your skin, hair, and nails work tirelessly to protect you, but the demands of modern living can take a toll. Prolonged exposure to sunlight, particularly UV rays, can disrupt the natural balance of your skin. Combat these effects by incorporating skincare products enriched with protective ingredients designed to minimize environmental stressors. Extend the care to your hair and nails by practicing thoughtful habits. Clean your nail tools regularly to maintain hygiene, protect your scalp from the sun with hats, and use gentle, nourishing hair products to support health and vitality. These small yet impactful steps are a meaningful way to preserve your natural beauty and ensure your appearance thrives for years to come.

Hair, Nail, and Skin Care Preservation

Nourishing your skin, hair, and nails is like cultivating a garden. What you feed the soil determines the health and vitality of every leaf, strand, and nail. These essential elements thrive on a diet rich in omega-3 fatty acids, biotin, vitamins A, C, and E, and minerals like zinc. Each avocado, salmon fillet, and a handful of nuts is more than just a meal; it's a gift to your skin's glow, your hair's strength, and your nails' resilience. Eating well is like building a fortress of vitality from the inside out, preserving the radiance of your appearance against the wear and tear of time.

Dry patches, brittle nails, or sudden hair thinning are cues from your body, signals that it's time for extra attention. Keeping an eye on these subtle signs is a way of listening to what your body needs, just as maintaining a good skincare routine and up-to-date haircare and nailcare practices are like arming yourself with powerful allies. In the end, our skin, hair, and nails aren't just parts of us; they're precious indicators of our health and well-being. Embracing a lifestyle that prioritizes their care is more than maintenance. It is an expression of self-respect. From feeding our bodies with nutrients to casting away harmful habits and staying active, each step is a commitment to preserving the beauty and strength of these natural assets.

As we wrap up this journey through the ins and outs of hair, nail, and skincare, remember: your beauty routine is more than skin-deep! By taking these simple steps to prevent, protect, and preserve, you're not just giving your appearance a boost. You are investing in lifelong health and vitality. Every sunscreen application, nutritious snack, and regular check-up is like adding a layer of armor to keep you looking and feeling your best. So, next time you slather on that moisturizer or take a break from screen time, know that you're doing more than just pampering yourself. You're setting the stage for healthier skin, stronger hair, and resilient nails that will thank you for years to come. Cheers to a glow that lasts and a future full of good hair days, clear skin, and nails that can handle whatever life throws at them!

As we bring this bonus wellness chapter to a close, "The 360° Health Care Plan: From Prevention to Protection to Preservation," we're reminded of the incredible power of proactive self-care. From regular check-ups and lab tests that catch early warning signs to intentional practices that protect and preserve our health, each step we take builds a foundation for lifelong wellness. Whether it's safeguarding our vision, nurturing our skin, or cherishing the resilience of our hair and nails, these small but impactful actions help us embrace the fullness of life with confidence. Let this chapter inspire you to make every choice a step toward a healthier, brighter, and more vibrant you.

Take Action: Schedule your Dermatology Exams

YEAR	DATE	TIME	DOCTOR

RESOURCES

CONTACT AND CONNECT

SERAPHIM MEDICAL, LLC

connect@seraphimmed.com

@seraphimmedspa

@drtinillejenkins.com

[Sleep Relaxation](https://www.youtube.com/watch?v=6DwCP4GQlEo)
(https://www.youtube.com/watch?
v=6DwCP4GQlEo)

OTHER LITERARY WORKS

Grab my parent's book. It includes 7 other couple's stories including a prisoner of war…

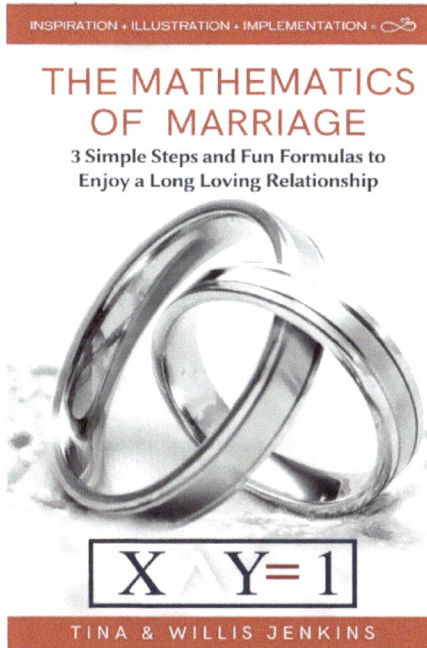

INSPIRATION + ILLUSTRATION + IMPLEMENTATION = ∞

THE MATHEMATICS OF MARRIAGE

3 Simple Steps and Fun Formulas to Enjoy a Long Loving Relationship

$X \wedge Y = 1$

TINA & WILLIS JENKINS

MathofMarriage.com

Grab my grandmother's autobiography…

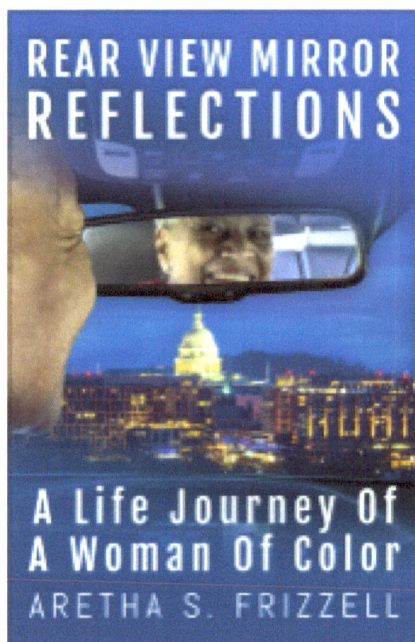

REAR VIEW MIRROR
REFLECTIONS

A Life Journey Of
A Woman Of Color

ARETHA S. FRIZZELL

Arethafrizzell.com

Dr. Tinille T. Jenkins, DMS, P.A-C, MSMS, CLS (ASCP)

www.ingramcontent.com/pod-product-compliance
Lightning Source LLC
Chambersburg PA
CBHW040512290326
41930CB00035B/3